THE ATKINS DIET
(A Beginner's Practical Guide):

A Comprehensive Quick-Start Guide to Shredding Weight and Feeling Great: A 14 Day Diet Plan for a Simple Start (Atkins for beginners, Atkins……, Atkins

By

ROBB SMITH

Copyright © 2019, by: ROBB SMITH

ISBN-13: 978-1-950772-17-9

ISBN-10: 1-950772-17-9

All Rights Reserved. No part of this publication may be reproduced in any form or by any means, including scanning, photocopying, or otherwise without prior written permission of the copyright holder.

Disclaimer:

The information provided in this book is designed to provide helpful information on the subjects discussed. The publisher and author are not responsible for any specific health or allergy needs that may require medical supervision and are not liable for any damages or negative consequences from any treatment, action, application or preparation, to any person reading or following the information in this book.

Table of Contents

- INTRODUCTION 5
- THE NEW ATKINS DIETING MADE EASY 5
- SUMMARY ON THE "DO'S AND DONT'S" DURING THE FOUR PHASES OF THE ATKINS DIET 5
- Twisted Tuna Salad 9
- Fish Tacos Recipe 10
- Cherry tomato salsa 12
- Balsamic vinaigrette 13
- Paleo Chicken Fajitas 14
- Liver & onions 15
- Bacon, spinach & mushroom casserole 16
- Chicken & zucchini hot salad 17
- Sausages with parsnip mash & mushrooms 19
- Crockpot Breakfast Casserole 21
- Sour Cream & Bacon Crock Pot Chicken 23
- Slow Cooker Chipotle Barbacoa Brisket 25
- Slow Cook Thai Chicken 27
- Crock Pot Balsamic Roast 29
- Rosemary Lemon Garlic Lamb with Sweet Potato Noodles 31
- Slow Cooker Chicken Roll-Ups with Prosciutto and Asparagus 33
- Slow-Cooker Korean-Style Beef Short Ribs 35
- CROCK POT SWISS STEAK 37
- Turkey Avocado Cobb Salad 39
- Greek Salad 40
- Grilled Chicken Caesar Salad 41
- Chicken Caesar 42
- CROCK POT CASHEW CHICKEN 43
- Crockpot Chicken de Provence 44
- Honey-mustard Drumsticks Recipe 45
- Spicy Sriracha Chicken Wings Recipe 46
- Slow Cooked Bacon-Wrapped Chicken Recipe 47
- Turkey Chili Recipe 48
- Kansas City BBQ Wings Recipe 50
- Barbecued Sirloin in Dijon Recipe 51
- Cuban Shredded Beef Recipe 52
- Salmon with Cherry Tomato Salsa and Asparagus Recipe 54
- Easy Coronation chicken 55
- Summer Antipasto 56
- Toasted Almond Chicken Salad 58

- Scrambled Whites with Green 59
- Cinnamon and Apple Natural Muesli 60
- Bake Fish Recipe 61
- Chicken Fried Rice 63
- Club Sandwich 65
- Grilled Chicken with Mushroom Sauce 66
- Smashed Avocado on Toast 68
- Lemon Chili Chicken Salad 69
- Torte Del Re - King's Cake 71
- Pizza Frittata 72
- Berry Protein Shake 74
- Miraculous Brownies 75
- Blueberry Almond Breakfast Pudding 76
- Pasta with Chicken and Roasted Red Pepper Sauce 78
- Pasta Salad - Basil and Tomato Salad 79
- Strawberry Chicken Salad 80
- Pecan Nut Pie Crust 81
- Tofu Scramble 82
- Tangy Grilled Salmon 83
- Cranberry Walnut Cookies 84
- Dried Cranberries 86
- Garlic Parmesan Flax Seed Crackers 87
- Chopped Salad 88
- Almond Pie Crust 89
- Cherry Nut Cake 90
- Conclusion 91

INTRODUCTION

THE NEW ATKINS DIETING MADE EASY

The Atkins Diet was propounded in 1972 by a cardiologist Robert C. Atkins. The Atkins Diet is a popular low-carbohydrate eating plan that restricts on the excess intake of carbohydrates while emphasizing protein and fats.

Dr. Atkins made the derivation that there are crucial unrecognized factors in our eating habits that make us fat. He made us to understand that the major factor that makes us to put on much weight by the day is our consumption of refined carbs, especially sugar, high-fructose corn syrup, and flour.

The summary of the theory is that when you drastically cut back on carbs, your body turns to your fat stores for fuel. The result is you burn body fat, releasing a by-product which is called ketones, that you will use for energy.
The thrust of the Atkins Nutritional Approach is to reduce one's carbohydrate (carbs) intake and increase once intake of protein and fat.
According to Dr. Atkins' New Diet Revolution 1, which stipulates that diet, which is low in carbs, triggers a metabolic advantage; the body burns more calories than it would on other diets. Nevertheless, during this metabolic advantage, the body also gets rid of some unused calories.

The Atkins diet is made up of four-phase eating program, which is combined with vitamin and mineral supplements, as well as regular exercise.

SUMMARY ON THE "DO'S AND DONT'S" DURING THE FOUR PHASES OF THE ATKINS DIET

Tips:

As you kick-start with the stages in the Atkins diet, I will recommends you do at least 30 minutes of exercise on most days of the week.

2.1. THE FIRST PHASE (INDUCTION PHASE):

1. The first phase of the Atkins diet may be challenging, due to the limited list of foods you expected to eat. This will require you to skip many of your favorite foods and treats.

2. It is during this phase that your body switches from burning carbs to burning fat and stabilizes the blood sugar levels and you end up losing 6-10lb in a week.

3. This phase last for duration of two (2) weeks and you expected to eat just 20 grams of net carbs daily.

4. Make sure you drink about eight (8) glasses of water daily.

WHAT TO EAT DURING THE PHASE ONE OF THE ATKINS DIET

1. PROTEIN AND FATTY FOOD: such as poultry, cream, eggs, fish, shellfish, red meat, cream, butter, and vegetable oils

2. VEGETABLES: such as broccoli, asparagus, cucumber, celery, green beans and peppers,

WHAT YOU SHOULDN'T EAT DURING THE INDUCTION PHASE OF THE ATKINS DIET

AVOID FOODS LIKE fruits, biscuits, cakes, chocolate, crisps, starchy vegetables, fizzy drinks, croissants, rice, pastry sugary baked goods, breads, milk, pastas, potatoes, grains, nuts, seeds or alcohol.

THE SECOND PHASE (BALANCING PHASE OR ON- GOING WEIGHT LOSS):

1. In this phase, you take a total of 25g-50g of carbohydrate daily to lose between 1 and 3lb a week.

2. In this stage, you allowed to eat nutrient-rich carbs, such as vegetables, seeds, nuts, legumes, berries and other fruit, wine and other low-carb alcohol, and whole grains as you continue to lose weight.

3. You also continue to avoid foods such as Bread, potatoes, rice, pasta and breakfast cereals.

4. I suggest you stay in this phase until you are about 10 pounds (4.5 kg) from your weight loss goal.

THE THIRD PHASE (PRE-MAINTAINANCE):

Note: you only start this phase once you have just 5-10lb left to lose
1. In this phase, you gradually increase the range of foods you eat, including fruits, porridge, bread, pasta, starchy vegetables and whole grains.

2. I suggest you add about 10 grams of carbs to your daily diet each week, but you need to keep a close eye on your weight and cut back if your weight loss stops.

3. The sole purpose of this phase is to slow down your weight loss to no more than 1lb a week in an effort to prepare your body for the final phase (weight maintenance).

4. I advise you stay in this phase until you reach your weight goal.

THE FOURTH PHASE (LIFE TIME-MAINTAINANCE):

NOTE: You are to embark on this phase only when you reach your goal weight, and then you continue this way of eating for life.
1. This phase aims at helping you maintain your weight.

2. In this phase, you are advice to eat 90g of carbohydrate daily.

2.5. Reason why you have to stick to the diet

If you effectively stick to the Atkins diet, you will not only lose weight but will also keep it off.

The most troubling problem among Atkins dieter is that they drop out of the diet, as they do with most other diets. Study after study has discovered that after two or three years, the vast population of people who started well on the Atkins diet did not continue long-term. In the medium-term the

Atkins Diet tends to fare much better than other diet
Researchers at Stanford University carried out a study and found that people following the Atkins diet had best blood pressure levels, better cholesterol levels, disease prevention and lost and maintain the most weight, compared to people on other diets.

Atkins Diet shields the body from obesity and related health problems, such as type-2 diabetes and heart disease.

The Atkins Diet does not require counting calorie or portion control, all it requires of you is to keep track on your daily carbs consumption.

THE 14 DAY ATKINS DIET PLAN FOR A NEW YOU

Twisted Tuna Salad

Ingredients
½ cup of carrot, finely chopped
½ cup of parsley, finely chopped
4 finely chopped scallions
½ cup plus 2 Tablespoons of mayonnaise
10 to 12 turns of black pepper, freshly ground
4 (5-ounce) cans of solid white albacore tuna (in water), drained very well
½ cup celery, finely chopped
⅓ Cup of red onion, finely chopped
1 small clove garlic (crushed)
1 teaspoon of kosher salt

Directions:
1. First, you drain the canned tuna very well.
2. After which you dump in to a large mixing bowl and set aside.
3. After that, you use the food processor with the chopping blade to process the following ingredients individually (carrot, celery, parsley, red onion and scallion.
4. Make sure you measure after chopping so you get the exact amount of each ingredient.
5. Then you add to bowl with tuna along with small clove garlic (crushed), mayonnaise, salt and pepper.
6. At this point, you use a fork to gently mash any very large chunks of tuna and then mix all the ingredients together.
7. Finally, you serve cold.

Nutrition Information
Amount per serving
Calories: 113.0
Fat: 2.5g
Protein: 17.2g
Dietary Fiber: 1.3g
Carbohydrates: 7.1g

Fish Tacos Recipe

Ingredients
2 tablespoons of Paleo cooking fat
8 cloves garlic (minced)
4 cups of tomatoes (diced)
6 tablespoons of lime juice
2 avocado (sliced)
2 lbs. of fresh tilapia fillets
2 medium onions (chopped)
2 or 4 jalapeño pepper(s) (finely chopped)
½ cup of fresh cilantro (finely chopped)
Sea salt and freshly cracked black pepper to taste

Directions:
1. First, you combine the cooking fat with the garlic and onions in a large skillet over a medium-high heat.

2. After which you cook for about 5 minutes, until the onions are soft and translucent in color.

3. After that, you add the tilapia fillets to the skillet.

4. At this point, you allow the fillets to cook for about 3 to 4 minutes on one side prior to flipping.

5. As the fish starts to cook through, you use a fork to break it apart into flaky pieces.

6. Then you add the jalapeno pepper, cilantro, tomatoes, and lime juice to the mix and then season with salt and pepper to taste.

7. Finally, you cook for about 5 minutes before removing from heat.

8. After which you serve the taco filling to your liking and garnish with fresh avocado slices.

Nutritional value:
Amount per serving size: 1
Calories: 255
Fat: 4.92
Dietary fiber: 5.9g
Protein: 23.06g

Cherry tomato salsa

Ingredients
4 cloves garlic (minced)
2 teaspoons of fresh lemon juice
½ teaspoons of sea salt
½ cup of fresh oregano (chopped)
1 cup of cherry tomatoes (quartered)
2 teaspoons of lemon zest
4 tablespoons of olive oil
Freshly cracked black pepper to taste

Directions:
1. First, you combine the garlic, lemon zest, lemon juice, olive oil, salt and pepper in a small bowl.

2. After which you whisk well.

3. After that, you add the cherry tomatoes.

4. At this point, you toss the mixture together.

5. Then you serve over the salmon once it is cooked.

Nutritional value:
Amount per serving size: 1(92g)
Calories: 19.6
Fat: 0.1g
Carbohydrate: 4.5g
Protein: 0.8g

Balsamic vinaigrette

Tips:
This recipe is a classic of Italian cuisine and acts as a proper marinade for meat and it is famous when drizzled on cooked vegetables.

Ingredients
2 crushed clove of garlic
4 teaspoons of Dijon mustard (it is optional)
Sea salt and freshly ground black pepper to taste
1 ¼ cup of balsamic vinegar
2 teaspoons of dried oregano
1 ¼ cups of extra-virgin olive oil

Directions:
1. First, you put all the ingredients in a jar that has a lid.

2. After which you close the lid tight and shake well to combine the entire ingredients.

Nutritional value:
Amount per serving size: 2 tablespoons (31.0g)
Calories: 90
Fat: 8.0g
Carbohydrate: 4.0g

Paleo Chicken Fajitas

Tips:
This recipe takes on the classic fajita meal and is just as delicious without the tortilla.

Ingredients
6 bell peppers
4 tablespoons of oregano, chili powder, cumin and coriander
Juice of 10 lemons
A Butter lettuce to serve
6 lbs. of chicken breast (cut in thin strips)
6 onions (sliced)
12 chopped garlic cloves
8 tablespoons of cooking fat (preferable, coconut oil, tallow or ghee)
Choice of toppings for this recipe: diced tomatoes, sliced avocados, sauerkraut, salsa, guacamole, fermented pickles, mayonnaise and/or salsa Verde

Directions:
1. First, you combine the chicken, bell peppers, onions, spices, garlic and lemon juice in a bowl and mix thoroughly.

2. If you are preparing ahead of time, I suggest you let marinate in the refrigerator for about 4 hours.

3. When you ready to cook, you should first heat a large skillet on medium heat and cook the whole preparation with the cooking fat until the chicken is cooked through and the onion and bell pepper are soft.

4. Then you put the hot chicken preparation in a large bowl and let the people prepare their own fajitas on top of lettuce leaves with their favorite toppings.

Nutritional value:
Amount per serving size: 1 fajita
Calories: 450
Fat: 17g
Carbohydrate: 35g
Protein: 43g

Liver & onions

Ingredients
10 large onions (sliced)
Salt and pepper to taste
8 large slices pork (or beef liver)
12 tablespoons of butter or lard

Directions:
1. First, you heat a large skillet over medium-low heat and add 10 tablespoons of the butter and the sliced onions.

2. After which you cook slowly, stirring often, for about 20 to 25 minutes, until the onions are really soft and caramelized.

3. Then near the end of the cooking process of the onions, you heat another pan over a medium-high heat and cook the liver with the rest of the cooking fat, for approximately 3 minutes on each side.

4. After that, you serve the liver topped with the delicious and creamy cooked onions.

5. It is great when served with a little bit of homemade salsa on the side.

Nutritional value:
Amount per serving size: 6 oz.
Calories: 211
Fat: 5.02gg
Carbohydrate: 11.94g
Protein: 28.61g

Bacon, spinach & mushroom casserole

Ingredients
3 big handfuls of fresh spinach (stems removed)
A large onion (chopped)
Salt and pepper to taste
2 ½ lbs. of good quality smoked bacon (cut into medium sized strips)
1 lb. of button mushrooms (sliced)
2 tablespoons of lard, butter or ghee
2 garlic cloves (minced)

Directions:
1. First, you heat a large casserole over a medium heat and cook the bacon, making sure it is still soft.

2. After which you add the onion and cook until soft, for about 5 minutes.

3. After that, you add the garlic and cook for about a minute, until fragrant.

4. At this point, you add the mushrooms and cook for another 8 minutes, until soft.

5. Then you add the spinach and butter, cover and let cook for another 4 minutes, stirring occasionally, until the spinach is well cooked.

6. Finally, you season with salt and pepper and serve.

Nutritional value:
Amount per serving size: 1(268g)
Calories: 400.2
Fat: 27.2g
Carbohydrate: 15.9g
Fiber: 2.4g
Protein: 24.1g

Chicken & zucchini hot salad

Ingredients
5 zucchinis (cut into cubes)
1 tablespoon of oregano
7 tablespoons of homemade mayonnaise
2 cloves garlic (minced very finely)
Salt and pepper to taste
2.5 lbs. of chicken breast (cut into cubes)
3 tablespoons of coconut oil, butter, ghee or lard
1 large onion (chopped)
2 lemons Juice
1 head romaine lettuce (washed and shredded)

Directions:
1. First, you heat a large pan over a medium-high heat and cook the chicken cubes until well-cooked then set aside

2. Then in the same pan and with the rest of the cooking fat, add the onion and cook until soft, for 5 minutes.

3. After which you add the zucchini cubes, and oregano and season with salt and pepper.

4. After that, you cook until the zucchini cubes are soft.

5. At this point, you mix the mayonnaise, lemon juice and garlic in a bowl.

6. Then you add the hot and cooked chicken, onion and zucchini to the mayonnaise preparation and mix thoroughly.

7. Finally, you add the romaine lettuce, mix thoroughly and serve in bowls.

8. This hot salad is amazing when topped with some fresh almonds.

Nutritional value:
Amount per serving size: 1 chicken breast
Calories: 350
Fat: 14g
Carbohydrate: 22g
Protein: 37g

Sausages with parsnip mash & mushrooms

Ingredients
4 garlic cloves (minced)
4 teaspoons of cooking fat
2 lbs. of button mushrooms
4 tablespoons of chopped fresh oregano
Salt and pepper
24 large good quality beef or pork sausages
4 lbs. of parsnip (coarsely chopped)
10 tablespoons of butter or ghee
1cup of coconut milk or heavy cream
Pinches of nutmeg

Directions:
1. First, you boil the parsnips for about 15 minutes, until soft.

2. After which you drain the water, and add half the butter, coconut milk or heavy cream, pinches of nutmeg and salt and pepper to taste.

3. After that, you mash thoroughly with a potato masher (Note: you can also use a food processor for convenience)

4. Then you reserve the mashed parsnips in the covered pot so they stay warm.

5. At this point, you heat a large skillet over medium heat and cook the sausages in a large skillet with the cooking fat for 15 minutes, turning occasionally.

6. Furthermore, you set the sausages aside and add the mushrooms to the already hot skillet with the other half of the butter.

7. After which you cook until well browned, for about 5 minutes.

8. After that, you add the chopped oregano.

9. Finally, you serve the mashed parsnips covered with the sausages, mushrooms and all the drippings.

Nutritional value:
Amount per serving size: 1(400g)
Calories: 330
Fat: 11.6g
Protein: 22.0g
Fiber: 9g

Crockpot Breakfast Casserole

Notes
I suggest you use a Crockpot liner sprayed with non - stick cooking spray for easy clean - up.

Ingredients
2 cups of milk
2 lbs. of sausage, browned and drained (or 2 lb. of bacon, cooked and crumbled) or use both
½ teaspoon of dry mustard (it is optional)
1 teaspoon of black pepper
2 green pepper, diced (it is optional)
2 dozen eggs
2 packages (64 oz.) of frozen hash brown potatoes
4 cups of cheddar cheese (or Colby jack, shredded)
1 teaspoon of salt
1 cup of green onions, diced (it is optional)

Directions:
1. First, you spray your Crockpot with no stick cooking spray or preferably, you use a slow cooker liner and spray it.

2. After which you layer frozen potatoes, bacon or sausage, onions (if you using), green pepper (if you using) and 2 cups of shredded cheese in the Crockpot in two or three layers.

3. After that, you sprinkle the remaining 2 cups of shredded cheese over the top evenly.

4. At this point, you beat the eggs, milk, dry mustard, salt and pepper together.

5. Then you pour the eggs mixture over the cheese evenly in the Crockpot.

6. Finally, you cook on low for about 7 to 8 hours or until eggs are set and thoroughly cooked before, you serve.

Nutrition Information
Amount per serving 1(193)
Calories: 334.8
Fat: 23.7g
Protein: 16.6g
Carbohydrates: 13.2g

Sour Cream & Bacon Crock Pot Chicken

Ingredients
16 boneless and skinless chicken breasts
1 cup of flour
16 bacon slices
2 cups of sour cream
4 (10 oz.) cans of roasted garlic cream of mushroom soup

Directions:
This recipe can be prepared in two ways:

1. First, you place the bacon in a large skillet and then you cook over medium- low heat until some of the fat is rendered.

2. You should make sure that the bacon is still pliable and not crisp.

3. After which you drain on paper towels, and if you use this method, reduce the flour to ¼ cup or do not cook the bacon and proceed with the recipe.

4. After that, you wrap one slice of bacon around each boneless chicken breast and place in a 4 - 5 quart Crockpot.

5. At this point, you combine condensed soups, sour cream, and flour in medium bowl, and mix with wire whisk to blend.

6. Then you pour over chicken.

7. Furthermore, you cover Crockpot and cook on low for about 6 – 8 hours until chicken and bacon are thoroughly cooked.

8. This is when you remove the chicken and beat the sauce with a wire whisk so it is very well blended.

9. Finally, you pour sauce over chicken.

Nutrition Information
Amount per serving 1(260)
Calories: 419

Fat: 27.1g
Protein: 33.3g
Dietary Fiber: 0.1g
Carbohydrates: 8.8g

Slow Cooker Chipotle Barbacoa Brisket

Ingredients:
1 to 2 cups of my Chipotle Adobo Sauce (or 6 chipotles from a can plus 6 tablespoons of sauce)
2 small white onions (diced)
4 teaspoons of oregano
4 bay leaves
2 (2.5 to 4 pound) beef brisket
4 cups of beef stock
6 large cloves of garlic
1 teaspoon of ground cloves
2 tablespoons of apple cider vinegar

Directions:
1. First, you make a liquid puree with all of your ingredients except the beef or the bay leaves.

2. After which you pour about a quarter of your liquid puree into the bottom of your slow cooker.

3. After that, you trim any excessive fat from your brisket and place it in your slow cooker fat cap side down.

4. Remember that you do not need a lot of fat on your brisket at all.

5. At this point, you pour the rest of your liquid puree over your brisket ensuring that you coat the top sides.

6. Then you cook on low for about 8 hours.

7. Furthermore, you remove your brisket to a large bowl or container to pull/shred with 2 forks.

8. After which you add some of the cooking liquid from the crock-pot to your pulled brisket.

9. Serve in lettuce wrap tacos, with your eggs, over salads, or just by pulling strips off and feeding your face!

Nutrition Information
Amount per serving 1(272)
Calories: 362.2
Fat: 17.5g
Protein: 48.7g
Dietary Fiber: 0.3g
Carbohydrates: 2.6g

Slow Cook Thai Chicken

Ingredients:
1 large red bell pepper (seeded and sliced into strips)
½ cup of chicken broth
1 tablespoon of ground cumin
½ teaspoon of red pepper flakes
2 tablespoons of cornstarch
1 tablespoon of soy sauce
3 green onions (chopped)
½ cup of peanuts, chopped roasted
6 skinless, boneless chicken breast halves (cut into ½-inch strips)
1 large onion (coarsely chopped)
¼ cup of soy sauce
3 cloves of garlic (minced)
Salt and pepper
2/3 cup of creamy peanut butter
¼ cup of lime juice
¼ cup of chopped fresh cilantro

Directions:
1. First, you place the chicken breast strips, bell pepper and onion into a slow cooker.

2. After which you pour in the chicken broth and ¼ cup of soy sauce.

3. After that, you season with cumin, garlic, red pepper flakes, salt and pepper.

4. Then you stir to blend, then cover and cook on low for about 4 ½ to 5 hours.

5. At this point, you remove 1 cup of the liquid from the slow cooker, and mix this with the cornstarch, peanut butter, 1 tablespoon of soy sauce and lime juice.

Note: it should blend into a thick sauce.
6. Then you stir the sauce back into the slow cooker, and place the lid on the pot.

7. Finally, you cook on high for about 30 minutes.

8. Before serving make sure, you garnish with green onions, cilantro and peanuts.

Nutrition Information
Amount per serving 1(216g)
Calories: 388.9
Fat: 23.7g
Protein: 35.8g
Dietary Fiber: 3.5g
Carbohydrates: 11g

Crock Pot Balsamic Roast

Ingredients
4 lb. of top round roast
16 ounces tomato sauce
1 cup of water
4 tablespoons of coconut oil
Salt and Black Pepper, to taste
Garlic Powder
Balsamic Roast
2 large sweet onions (sliced)
1cup of balsamic vinegar
4 tablespoons of white wine
Rub
Smoked Paprika
Onion Powder

Directions:
1. First, you season your roast on both sides generously with the spices listed above to your desired amount.

2. After which you heat your coconut oil in a large pan over medium-high heat, and once it warm sear each side of your roast for 3-4minutes.

3. After that, you place your sliced onions in the bottom of your crock-pot and put your seared meat on top of the onions.

4. At this point, you combine your balsamic vinegar and tomato sauce in a bowl and mix thoroughly, and then pour over your meat in the crock-pot.

5. Then you add your water and white wine to your pan and de-glaze it.

6. Finally, you pour this mixture in your crock-pot as well and then place the lid on, set to low and cook for 6-8 hours.

7. After which you serve and enjoy!

Nutrition Information
Amount per serving 1(7 ounce)

Calories: 282
Protein: 36g
Carbohydrates: 2g

Rosemary Lemon Garlic Lamb with Sweet Potato Noodles

Tips:
Remember to save the bone from your leg of lamb that you can freeze and then use to make lamb stock.

Ingredients
6-8 stalks of fresh rosemary
Zest & juice of 2 lemons
4 medium sweet potatoes
4 tablespoons of olive oil
2-4 Tablespoons of flat leaf parsley, for garnish
1 leg of lamb
6-8 garlic cloves (peeled)
½ cup of liquid (either water or broth)
2-4 Tablespoons of ghee (or coconut oil)
Sea salt and black pepper, to taste

Directions:
1. First, you place your half leg of lamb fat side up onto a chopping board.

2. After which you use a sharp knife score the fat on top of the lamb in a crosshatch form.

3. After that, you season the lamb all over with sea salt & cracked black pepper.

4. At this point, you remove the rosemary from the stalk and add to a food processor, along with your lemon zest and garlic cloves.

5. Then you process until mixed then slowly drizzle in your olive oil.

6. Furthermore, you spread the paste all over the lamb, making sure to get the paste into the places you scored with your knife.

7. After which you place lamb in your slow cooker and then pour over ½ cup of liquid and squeeze over the juice of the lemon you zester.

8. After that, you place on low heat and allow cooking for about 6-8 hours.

9. Finally, once it is ready, you carefully remove to a chopping board and let rest for 10 minute before slicing/shredding.

Directions for the sweet potato noodles
1. First, you peel your sweet potatoes and then cut each one in thirds.

2. After which you use a spiraliser or a julienne peeler to create "noodle" strands.

3. At a point when your noodles are ready, you add your butter/ghee into a skillet and place on medium heat.

4. Then once melted, you throw in your noodles and season with S&P.

5. After that, you toss to coat and cook until softened.

6. Finally, you serve with some sliced slow cooked leg of lamb on top and garnish with some flat leaf parsley on top.

Nutrition Information
Amount per serving ()
Fat: 28g
Protein: 38g
Dietary Fiber: 3g

Slow Cooker Chicken Roll-Ups with Prosciutto and Asparagus

Ingredients:
12 to 16 slices of Prosciutto or spiced ham of choice (usually about a ½ pound will do)
Salt and Pepper to taste
6 or 8 boneless chicken breasts
2 bunches of asparagus
Garlic cloves

Directions:
1. First, filet your chicken breasts in ½.

2. After which you mash your chicken flat with a meat maillot or rather using a piece of saran wrap between the chicken and mallet helps.

3. You should smash the chicken on both sides until it is tenderized and ready to roll.

4. After that, you trim your asparagus spears to your desired length for your rolls.

5. Remember that cutting off about ½ the stalk usually works fine.

6. At this point, you place 6 to 8 pieces of asparagus along with 2 chopped cloves of garlic inside your chicken.

7. Then you proceed to roll up the chicken around the asparagus.

8. Furthermore, you roll a piece of Prosciutto or ham around your chicken roll up and you are ready to go. Make use of a wooden toothpick to hold your roll together is optional and is normally only necessary if you made a rather messy roll-up. By so doing everything will bind together nicely in the cooking stages.

10. Finally, you line the bottom of your slow cooker with the roll-ups and cook on low for about 4 hours.

Nutrition Information
Amount per serving 1(291g)
Calories: 855.1
Fat: 52.0g

Protein: 82.4g
Dietary Fiber: 4.7g
Carbohydrates: 14.5g

Slow-Cooker Korean-Style Beef Short Ribs

Ingredients:
2 onions (thinly sliced)
4-inch knob of fresh ginger (sliced)
1 rice wine vinegar
2 teaspoons of red pepper flake
Sea salt and pepper to taste
6 pounds of grass fed beef short ribs
6 cloves of garlic (minced)
1 cup of organic wheat free tamari (soy sauce or coconut aminos)
½ cup of raw honey
4 teaspoons of sesame oil
1 cup of chopped scallion

Directions:
1. First, you mix the tamari, rice wine vinegar and honey in the bottom of your slow cooker.

2. After which you add the sliced onion, garlic, ginger and red pepper flake to the slow cooker.

3. After that, you season your short ribs with sea salt and pepper.

4. At this point, you place them in the slow cooker and cook on high for about 3-4 hours or low for 6-8 hours.

5. At a point when the short ribs are cooked, you remove the bones and shred the beef.

6. Then you add it back into the slow cooker.

7. Finally, you stir in the sesame oil, taste and season if necessary.

8. After which you garnish with chopped scallion and serve.

Nutrition Information
Amount per serving 1(335g)

Calories: 1212.6
Fat: 111.6g
Protein: 45.2g
Dietary Fiber: 0.4g
Carbohydrates: 4.0g

CROCK POT SWISS STEAK

INGREDIENTS
½ cup of Arrowroot Starch
2 teaspoons of Sage
4 teaspoons of Salt
8 Carrots (peeled)
2 Medium Onion (sliced)
6 cups of Crushed Tomatoes (or preferably one 28 oz. can)
4 Tablespoons of Cooking Fat (lard, coconut oil, or ghee)
4 lbs. of Beef Round
4 teaspoons of Mustard Powder
2 teaspoons of Thyme Leaves
1 teaspoon of Black Pepper
8 Celery Stalks
6 Garlic Cloves (minced)
6 Tablespoons of Worcestershire Sauce

Directions:
1. First, you cut the beef into large pieces, about 3" cubes.

2. After which you combine the arrowroot starch and spices.

3. After that, you cut the carrots and celery into 3" long pieces and heat the cooking fat in a frying pan.

4. At this point, you coat the beef pieces with the spiced powder and pan fry until brown.

5. Then you transfer the meat into the crock-pot and add the carrots, celery, onions and garlic to the fry pan and then stir-fry for about 2-3 minutes until onions are mostly translucent.

6. This is when you transfer the vegetables to the crock-pot and turn off the heat in the frying pan.

7. After which you add the tomatoes and Worcestershire sauce to the frying pan to deglaze the leftover bits.

8. Then you transfer it all into the crock-pot.

9. Finally, you cover the crock-pot and cook on low for at least 8 hours.

Nutrition Information
Amount per serving 1(344g)
Calories: 364.6
Fat: 9.1g
Protein: 53.6g
Dietary Fiber: 2.2g
Carbohydrates: 14.5g

Turkey Avocado Cobb Salad

Ingredients:
2 tablespoons of olive oil
4 tablespoons of cider vinegar
16 cups of baby spinach leaves
A ripe avocado (cut into ½" cubes)
2 oz. blue cheese (crumbled)
2 lbs. of turkey breast cutlets
½ teaspoon of salt
2 teaspoons of Dijon mustard
8 slices of cooked reduced sodium turkey bacon, crumbled
8 cherry tomatoes (halved)

DIRECTIONS:
1. First, you preheat grill pan on medium high heat for about 2 minutes.
2. After which you brush turkey with 2 teaspoons of the oil and sprinkle with half of the salt.
3. After that, you grill turkey for about 4 minutes, flip, and continue cooking until centers are opaque and juices run clear, about 3 minutes longer.
4. Then you cut into chunks.

DIRECTIONS ON HOW TO PREPARE THE DRESSING:
1. First, you combine vinegar, mustard, 2 tablespoons of water, and remaining 4 teaspoons oil and ¼-teaspoon salt in glass jar.
2. After which you shake thoroughly.
3. Then you toss the spinach with 4 tablespoons of the dressing in large bowl.
4. At this point, you arrange turkey, bacon, avocado, tomatoes, and cheese over spinach.
5. Finally, you drizzle remaining dressing over salad and season with black pepper to taste.

Nutrition Information
Amount per serving
Calories: 288
Fat: 13.4g
Protein: 34g
Dietary Fiber: 5g
Carbohydrates: 10g

Greek Salad

Ingredients:
One green pepper (sliced)
One cucumber (sliced)
Feta cheese (crumbled)
Grilled chicken or preferably fish (it is optional)
One head romaine lettuce (or you substitute your favorite lettuce)
2 ripe tomatoes (sliced)
Thinly sliced red onion (as many as you want)
Kalamata olives (as many as you want)
One handful toasted pine nuts
Dressing
One tablespoon of fresh lemon juice
Pinch of oregano
4 Tablespoons of olive oil
One tablespoon of red wine vinegar
One slice fresh garlic (chopped or minced)
Salt and pepper to taste

Directions:
1. First, you clean, slice, and combine salad ingredients.
2. After which you mix dressing ingredients in a bowl, stirring with a fork, and give it the sniff test (if it smells too much of vinegar, I suggest you add more oil).
3. After that, you add to salad ingredients.
4. Then you toss and serve.
5. Enjoy!

Nutrition Information
Amount per serving
Calories: 395
Fat: 33.5g
Protein: 8g
Dietary Fiber: 7g
Carbohydrates: 17.5g

Grilled Chicken Caesar Salad

Tips:
This recipe is far lighter, and just as good, as the popular full- fat version.

Ingredients
2 teaspoons of canola oil
Freshly ground pepper, to taste
2 cups of fat-free croutons
Lemon wedges
2 pounds boneless, skinless chicken breasts, trimmed of fat
½ teaspoon of salt (or to taste)
16 cups washed, dried and torn romaine lettuce
1 cup Caesar Salad Dressing
1-cup Parmesan curls

Directions:
1. First, you prepare a grill or preheat broiler.
2. After which you rub chicken with oil and season with salt and pepper.
3. After that, you grill or broil chicken until browned and no trace of pink remains in the center, for about 3 to 4 minutes per side.
4. At this point, you combine lettuce and croutons in a large bowl, then toss with Caesar Salad Dressing, and divide among plates.
5. Then you cut chicken into 1/2-inch slices and fan over salad.
6. Finally, you top with Parmesan curls and then serve immediately, with lemon wedges.

Note:
1. To make parmesan curls, I suggest you start with a piece of cheese that is at least 4 ounces.
2. Make sure you use a swivel-bladed vegetable peeler to shave off curls.

Nutrition Information
Amount per serving
Calories: 278
Fat: 6g
Protein: 34g
Dietary Fiber: 1g
Carbohydrates: 14g

Chicken Caesar

Ingredients:
3 Tablespoons of grated Parmesan cheese
½ teaspoon of anchovy paste
½ teaspoon of Worcestershire sauce
6 cups of torn romaine lettuce
24 croutons (fat-free)
¼ cup of canola oil mayonnaise
2 Tablespoons of lemon juice
½-clove garlic (minced)
⅛ Teaspoon of black pepper
2 cups of cubed cooked boneless skinless chicken breast

Directions:
1. First, you combine the mayonnaise, Parmesan, lemon juice; anchovy paste, garlic, Worcestershire sauce, and pepper in a bowl and then mix well.
2. After which you combine the lettuce, chicken, and croutons in a separate bowl.
3. After that, you pour in the mayonnaise mixture and toss well to coat.
4. Then you divide among 4 bowls and serve.

Nutrition Information
Amount per serving
Calories: 278
Fat: 15g
Protein: 25g
Dietary Fiber: 1.5g
Carbohydrates: 8.5g

CROCK POT CASHEW CHICKEN

INGREDIENTS
1 cup of soy sauce
½ cup of ketchup
Four cloves garlic (minced)
½ teaspoon of red pepper flakes
½ cup of water
4 pounds boneless, skinless chicken thighs
½ cup of rice vinegar
4 tablespoons of brown sugar
2 teaspoons of fresh ginger, grated
1 cup of cashews
4 tablespoons of cornstarch

Directions:
1. First, you place chicken in crock-pot.

2. After which you combine soy sauce, vinegar, ketchup, sugar, garlic, ginger, and pepper flakes in small bowl.

3. After that, you mix well and pour over chicken.

4. Then you cook on low for about 3 to 4 hours or more.

5. When it is about 30 minutes before serving, you combine the water and cornstarch and add to the chicken.

6. Stir well and then you let the sauce thicken for the remainder of the cooking time.

7. Add cashews and stir just before serving.

8. Make sure you serve over rice.

Nutrition Information
Amount per serving size ¾ cups
Calories: 333
Fat: 12.7g
Protein: 69.0g
Dietary Fiber: 1g
Carbohydrates: 19g

Crockpot Chicken de Provence

Ingredients:
60 button mushrooms
2 Family packs of chicken thighs, remove skin (feel free to substitute with chicken breasts, drumsticks or pork chops)
2 dashes of sea salt and pepper, to taste
4 extra-large handfuls of Okra
8 tablespoons of minced garlic
2 jar of marinara sauce (or large can of tomato sauce)
6 tablespoons of herbs de Provence

Directions:
1. First, you place chicken thighs at the bottom of the Crockpot.

2. After which you season with salt and pepper.

3. After that, you cut the tops of the okra, put them in the Crockpot and sprinkle the okra with garlic.

4. At this point, you throw the mushrooms on top of the okra.

5. Then you pour your favorite clean marinara sauce on everything.

6. This is when you sprinkle the herbs de Provence on top.

7. Finally, when you done you put the Crockpot on low for about 8 hours or high for 4.

Nutrition Information
Amount per serving 1(446g)
Calories: 905
Fat: 68.3g
Protein: 63.6g
Dietary Fiber: 0.9g
Carbohydrates: 5.1g

Honey-mustard Drumsticks Recipe

Ingredients
½ cup of Dijon (or homemade mustard)
6 cloves garlic (minced)
4 tablespoons of coconut aminos (it is optional)
Sea salt and freshly ground black pepper to taste
8 lbs. of chicken drumsticks (washed and patted dry)
4 tablespoons of mustard powder
2/3 cup of raw honey (it is optional)
Chives for garnishing

Directions:
1. First, you whisk together the Dijon mustard, mustard powder, honey, garlic, coconut aminos, and salt, and pepper to taste in a small bowl.

2. After which you pour the mustard marinade over the drumsticks and refrigerate them for at least 2 hours.

3. Meanwhile, you heat your grill to a medium-high.

4. At this point, you grill the drumsticks for about 25 to 30 minutes, turning every 5 minutes and basting with any leftover marinade.

5. Finally, when the chicken is cooked, you then sprinkle with fresh chives and serve

Nutrition Information
Amount per serving 1(186g)
Calories: 301
Fat: 13.0g
Protein: 29.7g
Dietary Fiber: 0.5g
Carbohydrates: 15g

Spicy Sriracha Chicken Wings Recipe

Ingredients
2 teaspoons of garlic powder
2 tablespoons of fresh cilantro leaves, minced
4 lbs. of chicken wings
Sea salt and freshly ground black pepper, to taste
Ingredients for the Sriracha-based sauce
½ cup of raw honey (it is optional)
Juice of 2 limes
10 tablespoons of olive oil
½ cup of sriracha sauce
2 tablespoons of coconut aminos;

Directions:
1. Meanwhile, you heat your oven to a temperature of 400 F.

2. After which you combine the olive oil, honey, sriracha, coconut aminos, and lime juice in a small bowl.

3. After that, you combine the chicken wings, garlic powder, in a large bowl, and season with salt and pepper to taste.

4. At this point, you arrange the wings on a parchment paper covered baking sheet and bake for about 25-30 minutes, flipping them over halfway through.

5. Then you brush the wings with the Sriracha mixture and place them under the broiler for about 3-4 minutes, or until crisp and crusted.

6. Finally, you garnished with fresh cilantro and serve immediately.

Nutrition Information
Amount per serving 1(515)
Calories: 1720.1
Fat: 131.2g
Protein: 120g
Dietary Fiber: 2.0g
Carbohydrates: 7.8g

Slow Cooked Bacon-Wrapped Chicken Recipe

Ingredients
3 cups of homemade BBQ sauce
8 apples (peeled and chopped)
16 to 24 slices bacon
8 boneless skinless chicken breasts
4 tablespoons of fresh lemon juice
2 onions (diced)

Directions:
1. First, you wrap each chicken breast with bacon slices.

2. After which you place each bacon-wrapped chicken breast in your slow cooker.

3. After that, you combine the BBQ sauce, lemon juice, apples, and onions in a bowl, and mix thoroughly.

4. At this point, you pour the BBQ sauce mixture over the chicken.

5. Then you cover and cook on low for about 6 to 8 hours.

6. Finally, you serve the chicken breasts topped with the apple and onion mixture.

Turkey Chili Recipe

Ingredients
4 cups of carrots (sliced or diced)
4 bell pepper (chopped)
4 tablespoons of tomato paste
2 cups of chicken (or turkey stock)
2 tablespoons of ground cumin
2 teaspoons of dried oregano
Green onions, sliced (it is optional, for garnishing)
6 to 8 cups of shredded, cooked turkey meat
4 cups of onions (chopped)
4 cups of diced tomatoes
8 garlic cloves (minced)
4 tablespoons of chili powder or to taste
2 tablespoons of dried hot red pepper flakes
Paleo cooking fat
Sea salt and freshly ground black pepper to taste

Directions:
1. First, you melt some cooking fat in a large saucepan placed over a medium-high heat, and cook the onions, bell peppers and carrots for about 5 minutes until the onions are golden.

2. After which you add the garlic, chili powder, cumin, red pepper flakes, and oregano.

3. After that, you stir well and cook for a minute.

4. Then you add the tomato paste, diced tomatoes, chicken or turkey stock, cooked turkey meat, and season with salt and pepper to taste.

5. At this point, you give everything a good stir and then bring the chili to a simmer, reducing the heat to low, and let it simmer, uncovered, for about 30 to 45 minutes.

6. Make sure you serve warm with freshly sliced green onions on top.

Nutrition Information
Amount per serving 1(336g)
Calories: 310.6
Fat: 13.7g
Protein: 23.1g
Dietary Fiber: 8.5g

Kansas City BBQ Wings Recipe

Ingredients
Twenty chicken wings
Ingredients for the Kansas City BBQ sauce
3 garlic cloves (minced)
¼ cup of honey, it is optional
1½ tablespoons of chili powder
½ teaspoons of onion powder
Sea salt and freshly ground black pepper to taste
3 cups of homemade ketchup
¼ cup of apple cider vinegar
2 tablespoons of homemade Worcestershire sauce
1 teaspoons of smoked paprika
1 teaspoon of cayenne pepper

Directions:
1. Meanwhile, you heat your oven to a temperature of 425 F.

2. After which you combine all the ingredients for the Kansas City BBQ sauce in a bowl and season to taste with salt and pepper.

3. After that, you combine the chicken wings with the BBQ sauce, in a large bowl, and toss gently to coat.

4. Then you place the chicken wings on a baking sheet and line them up in a single layer.

5. Finally, you bake in the oven for approximately 20 to 25 minutes.

6. Make sure you serve warm.

Nutrition Information
Amount per serving (10.4 oz.)
Calories: 520
Fat: 25g
Protein: 75g
Dietary Fiber: 1g
Carbohydrates: 1g

Barbecued Sirloin in Dijon Recipe

Ingredients
4 tablespoons of fresh basil (coarsely chopped)
2 tablespoons of Dijon mustard
4 tablespoons of white wine vinegar
4 lbs. of beef sirloin
4 tablespoons of ground black pepper
2 tablespoon of extra-virgin olive oil;

Directions:
1. First, you combine the basil, the black pepper, the olive oil, the Dijon mustard and the white wine vinegar in a bowl.

2. After which you rub the marinade onto the sirloin and refrigerate for about 1½ hours.

3. Meanwhile, you heat the BBQ or grill to medium-high, and cook the sirloin for about 12 to 15 minutes on each side.

4. Finally, you let the meat rest around 15 minutes before serving.

Nutrition Information
Amount per serving 1(272g)
Calories: 493.0
Fat: 34.7g
Protein: 31.9g
Dietary Fiber: 0.6g
Carbohydrates: 4.5g

Cuban Shredded Beef Recipe

Ingredients
6 garlic cloves (minced)
1 teaspoons of ground cumin
1 teaspoon of lime zest
2 cups of beef stock
Lime wedges (for serving)
4 lbs. of boneless beef chuck
2 onions (thinly sliced)
4 tablespoons of fresh orange juice
2 tablespoons of lime juice
Cooking fat
Sea salt and freshly ground black pepper

Directions:
1. First, you season the beef all over with sea salt and black pepper to taste.

2. After which you place the beef in a slow cooker with the stock and cook for 6 to 8 hours on low.

3. After that, when the beef is cooked, break it apart gently with a fork and set aside.

4. At this point, you melt the cooking fat in a large skillet placed over a medium-high heat.

5. Then you add the garlic and onion, and cook for about 5 minutes until the onion is golden and soft.

6. Furthermore, you add the beef to the skillet.

7. After which you reduce the heat to medium and cook for about 4 minutes.

8. Then you add the cumin, orange juice, lime juice, lime zest, and season again with salt and pepper to taste.

9. Finally, you give everything a good stir and then serve warm with lime wedges.

Nutrition Information
Amount per serving 1(289g)
Calories: 715.3
Fat: 57.9g
Protein: 42.1g
Dietary Fiber: 0.4g
Carbohydrates: 4.9g

Salmon with Cherry Tomato Salsa and Asparagus Recipe

Ingredients
4 cloves garlic (minced)
1 teaspoon of freshly ground black pepper to taste
2 teaspoons of lemon zest
2 tablespoons of olive oil
8 wild salmon fillets (skin-on)
1 teaspoons of sea salt
1 teaspoons of paprika
2 teaspoons of fresh lemon juice

Directions:
1. First, you set your oven to broil.

2. After which you combine the garlic, salt, pepper, paprika, lemon zest, lemon juice and olive oil in a small bowl and whisk well.

3. After that, you rub the salmon thoroughly with the mixture on both sides.

4. Then you place in a covered dish to marinade in the refrigerator for about 35 minutes.

5. At this point, you line a baking sheet with foil and once the salmon has marinade, place on the baking sheet and place in the oven to broil for about 8 to 10 minutes, or until pale pink and flaky.

Nutrition Information
Amount per serving ()
Calories: 265
Fat: 12.6g
Dietary Fiber: 1.8g
Carbohydrates: 9.6g

Easy Coronation chicken

Tip:
Make sure you use half mayonnaise, half crème fraîche for a lower fat version of this recipe

Ingredients:
150g (6 oz.) mango chutney
2-dessert spoon lime zest
1000g (2 ½ lbs.) skinless, boneless chicken breast fillets (cooked and diced)
200g (8 oz.) mayonnaise
2 teaspoons of curry powder
1 teaspoon of salt
8 tablespoons of fresh lime juice

Directions:
1. First, you whisk together the mayonnaise, chutney; curry powder, lime zest, lime juice and salt in a large bowl.

2. After which you add chicken and toss with the dressing until well coated.

3. After that, you cover and chill until serving.

Nutrition Information
Amount per serving 1(185g)
Calories: 333.8
Fat: 15.9g
Protein: 32.2g
Dietary Fiber: 1.0g
Carbohydrates: 15g

Summer Antipasto

It is time to satisfy your Italian cravings with this almost no-cook, vegetable-heavy main dish.

Ingredients for the Dressing
4 tablespoons of olive oil
¼ teaspoon of dried basil
¼ teaspoon of ground black pepper
6 tablespoons of red wine vinegar (or balsamic vinegar)
1 clove garlic (minced)
¼ teaspoon of salt
Ingredient for the Salad
2 medium zucchini (cut into 2" matchsticks)
2 cups of cherry tomatoes, halved
2/3 cup of pitted kalamata olives, pitted
32 slices turkey pepperoni
2 small bunch broccolis (cut into florets)
2 lbs. shrimp (cooked)
1 cup of canned artichoke hearts (drained and quartered)
2 (4 oz.) part-skim mozzarella cheese (cut into ½" cubes)
16 slices reduced-fat deli ham (rolled into tubes)

DIRECTIONS ON HOW TO MAKE THE DRESSING:
First, you whisk the red wine or balsamic vinegar, oil, garlic, basil, salt, and black pepper in a small bowl.

DIRECTIONS ON HOW TO MAKE THE SALAD:
1. First, you bring a medium saucepan of water to a boil.
2. After which you fill a large bowl with ice water and set near the stove.
3. After that, working in batches, you boil the broccoli and zucchini just until tender (they will turn bright green).
4. At this point, you use a slotted spoon to transfer the vegetables to the ice water to halt the cooking process and then drain well.
5. Then you place the shrimp in the center of a large platter.
6. Finally, you arrange the broccoli, zucchini, tomatoes, artichoke hearts, olives, cheese, ham, and pepperoni in small mounds around the shrimp.
7. After which you drizzle with the dressing.

Nutrition Information
Amount per serving
Calories: 272
Fat: 13.5g
Protein: 30g
Dietary Fiber: 3g
Carbohydrates: 8g

Toasted Almond Chicken Salad

Ingredients:
6 ribs of celery (sliced)
1 cup of low-fat plain yogurt
3 teaspoons of dried tarragon
Ground black pepper, to taste
2 bags (10 oz.) mixed greens
6 small chicken breast halves
2 bunches chives (finely chopped)
½ cup of light sour cream
4 tablespoons of slivered almonds, toasted
Salt

Directions:
1. First, you coat a nonstick skillet with cooking spray and place over medium-high heat.
2. When it is hot, you add the chicken and cook for about 4 minutes per side, or until the juices run clear.
3. After that, you remove the chicken from the heat and let it rest for at least 10 minutes.
4. At a point, when they are cool enough to handle, you chop the chicken breasts into small pieces.
5. After which you combine the chicken, celery, chives, yogurt, sour cream, and tarragon in a large bowl and then mix lightly.
6. Finally, you cover and refrigerate for at least 1 hour, or up to 24 hours.
7. Then you add the almonds, and salt and pepper to taste and serve on a bed of greens.

Nutrition Information
Amount per serving
Calories: 177
Fat: 5g
Protein: 25g
Dietary Fiber: 3g
Carbohydrates: 8g

BONUS RECIPES TO HELP YOU THROUGH THE OTHER STAGES

Scrambled Whites with Green

Ingredients:
3 ounces cream cheese (cut into bits and softened)
Five large eggs
Five chopped scallions
2 tablespoon unsalted butter

Directions:
1. First, you cook the scallions in the butter in a small non-stick skillet, over a moderately low heat, stirring until they are soft.

2. After which you whisk together the egg, cheese, salt and pepper inside the bowl.

3. Then you pour the mixed egg into the skillet and cook over a moderate heat, stirring for 3 to 4 minutes, until it is cook through.

Nutritional value:
Serving size per 100g
Calories: 225
Fat: 25.0g
Carbohydrate: 4.0g
Protein: 14.8g

Cinnamon and Apple Natural Muesli

Ingredients:
2 tablespoons sultanas
Two tablespoons flake almonds
A teaspoon chia seeds
An apple (diced into little chunk)
½ cup rolled oats
4 tablespoon all bran sticks
Sprinkle in some cinnamon
½ cup of milk

Directions:
1. First, you put all the entire ingredients in a bowl, mix thoroughly.

2. After which you add milk and stir, leaving it for some minute until the milk soak into the oats.

3. After that, you add a drizzle of honey (optional).

4. Make sure you serve immediately.

Nutritional value:
Serving size per 100g
Calories: 122
Fat: 3.2g
Carbohydrate: 16.6g
Protein: 18.0g

Bake Fish Recipe

Ingredient:
A packet of rice noodles
½ cup of water
1 ½ fresh spinach (large packet)
2 ½ firm thick white snapper/barramundi fish fillets (500g)
A silver butter
Shower some sesame seeds marinade
A teaspoon chili paste
2 ½ teaspoons soy sauce, salt reduced
2 teaspoons mirin
One ½ teaspoons ginger/garlic /sesame oil/brown sugar/fish sauce

Tips:
1. Determine the cooking time by the thickness of the fish.

2. Heat your oven to 180c (350f).

Directions:
1. When the oven gets heated, you line a baking tray/dish with baking paper, placing the fish fillets on the paper.

2. Stir the marinade ingredients in a little bowl.

3. Coat half the top of the fish with the sauce, using a pastry brush and shower it with sesame seeds.

4. Put it for 15mins in the oven and cook.

5. After the 15mins of being in the oven take it out and drizzle the remaining sauce over the fish, which you further cook for 10mins.

6. In the meantime, boil water in the kittle, soak the noodles in a bowl using the boiling water, and drain.

7. Place the spinach in a large heated non-stick fry pan, add garlic and water, and stir until it wilts down to nearly nothing.

8. Use salt and pepper to season it and at the last minute add a silver butter and turn the heat off.

9. Make sure you serve immediately.

Nutritional value:
Serving size per 100g
Calories: 87
Fat: 2.8g
Carbohydrate: 5.0g
Protein: 9.8g

Chicken Fried Rice

Ingredients:
½ cup of water
A tablespoon hoi sin sauce
A tablespoon oyster sauce
A tablespoon olive oil
A tablespoon soy sauce, light
A small sliced onion
Two cups cooked rice
Two small chicken breasts (400g)
A cup broccoli cut into florets
½ small-diced capsicums
Eight small sliced mushrooms
A diced carrot
A cup of frozen peas/corn
Two eggs (whisked in a bowl using a fork)
A tablespoon crushed ginger
A tablespoon crushed garlic

Tips: Make sure you cook the rice as per instructed and set it aside

Directions:
1. First, you heat a non-stick fry pan.

2. Spray with a non-stick cooking spray, adding the whisked egg, you then cook until half omelets half scrambled then you put it on a plate and set it aside.

3. Heat the pan with olive oil after you might have wiped it. Add onions, capsicum and mix for some minute then you take it off on a plate and set it aside.

4. When the pan is fully heat, you add the chicken, stir-fry until it is brown, take the heat off and add to your onion/capsicum plate.

5. You now add your broccoli, carrot, and ½ cup of water to the pan and simmer putting on the lid for two minutes after that you remove the lid and simmer until water has nearly evaporated.

6. Add into the pan, mushrooms with onions, chickens, garlic, capsicum, ginger, peas/corn, then soy, hoi sin and oyster sauce.

7. Then you finally add the rice and egg, stir until it is well blended, season with cracked pepper

8. Add a splash of soy (optional)

9. Make sure you serve immediately

Nutritional value:
Serving size per 100g
Calories: 114
Fat: 2.9g
Carbohydrate: 9.0g

Club Sandwich

Ingredient:
4 tablespoons low fat yoghurt dressing
Two eggs
Two lettuces (30g each)
6 slices whole meal or bread (multigrain)
Two 97% fat free ham (50g each)
A large tomato, sliced
100g chopped BBQ chicken breast

Directions:
1. First, you toast the six slices of bread.

2. After which you use a non-stick fry pan to fry the egg (no oil).

3. After that, you flip the egg until you cook to your desired taste.

4. Then you use the yogurt dressing to spread on each slices of bread.

5. At this point, you place the chopped chicken, lettuce and tomato; you then slice on top the ham and egg.

6. Finally, cut into ½ with a toothpick for stability in each slice.

Nutritional value:
Serving size per 100g
Calories: 137
Fat: 2.9g
Carbohydrate: 11.4g
Protein: 14.6g

Grilled Chicken with Mushroom Sauce

Ingredient:
½-cup water
A little pepper for seasoning
½ cup chopped parsley
¼-cup cold water mixed with 2 teaspoons corn flour
½ diced onion
Two cloves garlic
½ cup red wine
A tablespoon Worcestershire sauce
Teaspoon Dijon mustard
A cup of chicken reduced stock salt.
Fettuccine (200g)
Eight button sliced mushrooms
Two chicken breasts, pound with mallet between cling film
A tablespoon olive oil

Tips: in the meanwhile, cook the sauce (as per instructed), fettuccine and Steam your broccoli

Directions:
1. First, in a non-stick fry pan, spray the pan with a little olive oil.

2. After which you cook the onions for about 5minutes on a medium heat until it softened.

3. After that, you add your garlic and stir, add your red wine and cook until there is no liquid remaining.

4. Then you add the water and mushrooms and simmer for about two minute, add the Worcestershire sauce and Dijon mustard and simmer for another 2 minutes.

5. At this point, you season with pepper adding the stock and parsley simmers for some minute, add the corn flour mixed with water, this will now thicken.

6. In addition, you spray your olive oil on the chicken or grilled on a BBQ/grilled pan which will take you 10minutes or there about.

7. Once the chicken is cooked take off the heat and rest for a minute, then across the width, you slice into six slices.

8. Finally, you serve with chicken on top of fettuccine, sprinkle the sauce over, and place the broccoli on side.

Nutritional value:
Serving size per 100g
Calories: 93
Fat: 2.4g
Carbohydrate: 5.6g
Protein: 10.4g

Smashed Avocado on Toast

Ingredients:
An avocado (cut into chunk)
2 tablespoons crumbled feta
Two sliced light rye sour dough bread
2-tablespoon low fat cottage cheese
Six mint leaves
Five quartered cherry tomatoes
A teaspoon basil paste
S & p to taste
Fresh lemon or lime juice (squeezed)

Tips: toast your bread lightly

Directions:
1. First, you place the chunked avocado in a bowl together with the chopped mint leaves and add tomatoes.

2. After which you squeeze the lemon or lime juice over.

3. After that, you season with s & p spread the basil paste lightly over toast followed by the cottage cheese, followed also by the avocado.

4. Then you place on top of the cottage cheese, and then crumble feta on top.

Nutritional value:
Serving size per 100g
Calories: 185
Fat: 9.8g
Carbohydrate: 16.3g
Protein: 6.2g
Sodium: 243mg

Lemon Chili Chicken Salad

Ingredients:
3 tablespoon of olive oil
2chicken breast
½ juiced lemon
A juiced lime
A clove crushed garlic
½ grated lemon rind
½ teaspoon chili (adjust to taste)
S & p to taste

Ingredients for your salad
50g half-small bag lettuce
Five button sliced mushrooms
½ sliced cucumber (slice on angle)
½ red capsicums
Six quartered cherry tomatoes

Directions:
1. You start by cutting the chicken into large strips (note that each chicken should produce about 3 long strips),

2. After which you put in a non-metallic bowl together with lemon/lime juice, rind, chili, garlic with a teaspoon of olive oil.

3. After that, you place in the fridge for about 30minute to marinate.

4. At this point, you grill chicken until fully cooked on the BBQ or Griddle pan on a high heat.

5. Then you put the chicken in a plate and cover with foil.

6. Finally, you fix salad on plate ready for cooked chicken, sprinkle with a tablespoon olive oil and vinegar and serve immediately.

Nutritional value:
Serving size per 100g
Calories: 121

Fat: 4.6g
Carbohydrate: 0.9g
Protein: 18.4g

Torte Del Re - King's Cake

Tips:
Meanwhile, you grease a spring form pan or 10" round cake pan.
After which you heat oven to a temperature of 325 F.

Ingredients:
4 cups of almond meal
2 teaspoons of vanilla
Zest and juice of two lemons
10 eggs (separated)
1 teaspoon of salt
2 teaspoons of almond extract
Artificial sweetener (equal to 2 ½ cups of sugar)

Directions:
1. First, you whisk the egg yolks until light in color.

2. After which you beat the rest of the ingredients except for the egg white, ending with the almond meal.

3. At this point, it will be very stiff.

4. Then you beat egg whites until it is at a soft peak.

5. After that, you combine 1/3 of the egg whites with the rest of the mixture in other to loosen it up.

6. Then you fold the rest of the egg whites in, and put in greased pan.

7. Finally, you bake for about 30 minutes until toothpick comes out clean.

8. Allow it to cool completely in pan.

Nutritional value:
Amount per serving size: each of 8 servings
Calories: 185
Carbohydrate: 2.5g
Dietary fiber: 3g
Protein: 9g

Pizza Frittata

Tips:
1. This recipe can be for any meal. I prefer to make it for a quick dinner and eat the leftovers for breakfast and/or lunch.

2. It goes with any type of pizza fixings you desire.

Ingredients:
2 Tablespoons of water (you can use milk, cream, or half and half as you want)
2 green peppers, medium (about 2 ½ inches X 2 ¾ inches), chopped
4 oz. pepperoni (chopped)
4 cloves of garlic
8 oz. of shredded mozzarella cheese
12 eggs
3 Tablespoons of olive oil
8 oz. of mushrooms (sliced)
2 teaspoons of oregano
Salt and peppers to taste
1 cup of pasta sauce (sugar-free)

Directions:
1. First, you heat the oil in large nonstick ovenproof skillet. After which you Sauté for approximately 5 minutes the green peppers, mushrooms, and pepperoni.
2. After that, you add garlic and cook for another minute.
3. Then you add oregano, salt, and pepper then stir well. At this point, you whisk eggs and liquid together, and then add more salt and pepper.
4. This is when you add mixture to pan.
5. Then you mix egg mixture as it cooks for about 2-3 minutes, so cooked "curds" distributes throughout it should be enough "body" to float some pasta sauce on the top.
6. After which you add the cheese. Then you put the frittata under the broiler to brown the top.
7. Finally, make sure you cook the eggs through, and then you turn the oven down to 300 and give it a couple of minutes more.

Nutritional value:
Amount per serving size: each of 6 serving
Calories: 344
Carbohydrate: 7g
Dietary fiber: 2g
Protein: 21g

Berry Protein Shake

Tips:
If you prefer a lighter shake, such as for a snack, then I suggest you substitute unsweetened almond milk, soymilk, or the coconut milk in cartons.

Ingredients:
2 scoop low carb protein powder (I prefer "Designer Protein" for my calculations), plain or vanilla
4 Tablespoons of Flax Seed Meal
Sweetener to taste (I prefer liquid forms of Splenda - no carbs)
1 cup of coconut milk (the type in cans)
2/3 cup of frozen berries (I prefer strawberries for the analysis)
2 cups of water (feel free to put less, that only if you want it thicker)

Directions:
It simple, all you have to do is to put everything in the blender and whiz it together.

Nutritional value:
Amount per serving size: each serving
Calories: 429
Carbohydrate: 11g
Dietary fiber: 6g
Protein: 24g

Miraculous Brownies

Tips:
1. Meanwhile, you heat oven to 350 F and grease a 9 X 13 pan.
2. If you prefer a more bittersweet brownie, cut down on the artificial sweetener.

Ingredients:
4 cups of erythritol (powdered, not granulated)
8 eggs (room temperature is best)
2 teaspoons of salt
4 cups of flax seed meal
¼ cup of cream
2 cups of artificial sweetener
2 cups of walnuts (it is optional)
½ lb. of butter (1 stick)
2 Tablespoons of vanilla
1 cup of cocoa
8 oz. unsweetened chocolate (melted)
½ cup of water
2 Tablespoons of baking powder

Directions:
1. First, you cream the butter until fluffy.
2. After which you add the erythritol to the butter and cream them together until fully incorporated.
3. After that, you add the vanilla and beat the eggs into the mixture, one at a time.
4. At this point, you add salt and cocoa, beat very well.
5. Then you add chocolate and beat until fluffy.
6. This is when you add the rest of the ingredients and mix well to incorporate.
7. Finally, you pour into a pan and bake for approximately 35 to 40 minutes until top springs back.
Note: You can also test to make sure they are ready by sticking a toothpick in the brownies. If it comes out clean, then you know they done)
8. Make sure you cool, then cut into 32 squares. (Note: They are better when left overnight)

Nutritional value:
Amount per serving size: each of 32 brownies
Calories: 107
Fat: 10g
Carbohydrate: 1g
Dietary fiber: 3g
Protein: 3g

Blueberry Almond Breakfast Pudding

Tips:
1. You can make this recipe with any berries or other additions as listed.

2. It should be microwave in less than 5 minutes.

3. Note: increase the almond meal up to 1 cup, add 2 Tablespoons of water, and cook a bit longer.

Ingredients:
4 Tablespoons of water
½ cup of blueberries (frozen)
½ cup of almond meal
2 eggs
Add Sweetener and flavoring to taste.

Directions:
1. First, you mix the almond meal, egg, and water in a microwave-safe bowl.
2. Place the microwave on high for about 45 seconds.
3. After which you move the cooked part of the pudding towards the center of the bowl.
4. After that, you add blueberries and/or any mix-ins you want.
5. At this point, you microwave for approximately 45-60 seconds or more, depending on mix-ins, (Note: frozen fruit will need even longer cooking, because it will cool down the pudding).
6. Finally, you stir and eat.

Tips on possible Additions
An unsweetened coconut
A small cubes of cream cheese (any fat level will be preferable)
A sugar-free jam or preserves
Fresh or frozen berries or any other fruits
Chopped nuts
A sugar-free maple or any other syrup
A peanut butter or any other nut butters

Nutritional value:
Amount per serving size: each serving (with blueberry)

Calories: 273
Carbohydrate: 6g
Dietary fiber: 5g
Protein: 13g

Pasta with Chicken and Roasted Red Pepper Sauce

Ingredients:
3 lbs. boneless skinless chicken (cut into cubes) NOTE: For 5 servings or less for fewer servings
Salt and pepper to taste
Basil (preferably fresh chopped)
A Low carb pasta (if you using shirataki noodles, I recommend four 8 ounce packages works well for 8 servings)
1 cup of onion (finely chopped)
A roasted Red Pepper Cream Sauce (see link bellow)

Directions:
1. First, you season the chicken with salt and pepper.
2. After which you Sauté' chicken and onions in a small quantity of oil until cooked through.
3. After that, you heat the Roasted Red Pepper Sauce through in a saucepan or in the microwave. Note: do not boil.
4. Then you rinse shiratake noodles in hot water (or you prepare other low carb pasta).
5. At this point, you cut with kitchen shears to desired length.
6. Finally, you toss ingredients together.
7. If you have fresh basil, this is the time to chop some of it up and add.

Nutritional value:
Amount per serving size: each of 5 servings
Calories: 302
Carbohydrate: 4g
Dietary fiber: 2.5g
Protein: 33g

Pasta Salad - Basil and Tomato Salad

Ingredients:
2 cups of basil, chopped
6 oz. of mozzarella cheese (cut into small cubes)
2 Tablespoons of extra-virgin olive oil
2 package of shirataki noodles (or other pasta) - this makes about 6 servings
2 medium tomatoes (chopped)
2 Tablespoons of capers

Directions:
1. First, you rinse the shirataki noodles very well in a hot water.
2. After which you leave the noodles hot when combining with the other ingredients (this will helps to blend the flavors a bit).
3. Then you cut the shirataki noodles into manageable lengths using kitchen shears.
4. Finally, you toss the entire ingredients together.

Nutritional value:
Amount per serving size: each serving
Calories: 130
Carbohydrate: 3g
Dietary fiber: 2g
Protein: 8g

Strawberry Chicken Salad

Tips:
1. This is a lovely, light, and different recipe, which I can recommend for a summer dinner salad.
2. Make sure you dress with strawberry vinaigrette dressing and have a real treat on a hot summer night.

Ingredients:
8 cups of lettuce, spinach, and/or arugula (fill it in a 2-quart mixing bowl)
¼ cup of toasted almonds, sliced or slivered (you can still use toasted pine nuts or sunflower seeds)
½ lb. of boneless skinless chicken breast (grilled or broiled)
2 cups strawberries (sliced)
2 oz. of feta cheese, crumbled (Parmesan can also be preferable)

Directions:
1. First, you toss the greens with ¼-cup strawberry vinaigrette or other oil and vinegar kind of salad dressing.
2. After which you arrange the rest of the ingredients on top of the greens.
3. For meal-sized salads, I suggest you distribute between two plates or bowls.

Nutritional value: (without dressing)
Amount per serving size: each serving
Calories: 319
Carbohydrate: 9g
Dietary fiber: 5.5g
Protein: 35g

Pecan Nut Pie Crust

Tips:
You can use this recipe for other custard/pudding fillings.

Ingredients:
2 Tablespoons of melted butter
2 Tablespoons of sugar equivalent from artificial sweetener
1 cup of pecan pieces, frozen

Directions:
1. First, you take the pecans out of the freezer and measure them into a food processor (note: you can use a blender, but make sure you did not blend them down too small).
2. After which you pulse the processor until the largest pieces are as big as lentils or split peas.
3. After that, you add the butter and the sweetener (I like the "liquid Splenda").
4. At this point, you blend until it is evenly mixed.
5. Then you dump it into a pie pan, and push with your fingers to cover the bottom and sides.
6. Make sure that it is the right consistency to mold the crust to the pie pan evenly.

Nutritional value:
Amount per serving size: whole crust
Carbohydrate: 4.5g
Dietary fiber: 10.5g
Protein: 10g

Tofu Scramble

Ingredients:
4 Tablespoons of nutritional yeast
4 teaspoons of low sodium tamari (or preferably, soy sauce)
¼ teaspoon of black pepper
1 bell pepper (diced)
4 slices of Fakin' Bacon i.e. tempeh bacon substitute (chopped small)
2 lbs. of firm tofu
1 teaspoon of turmeric
¼ teaspoon of cayenne pepper
2 stalks of broccoli (chopped very well)
2 teaspoons of canola oil (or any other mild-flavored oil)
1 onion (diced)

Directions:
1. First, you drain the tofu.
2. After which you cut it into pieces and put it into a small mixing bowl.
3. After that, you add the nutritional yeast, turmeric, tamari/soy sauce, cayenne and pepper.
4. At this point, you use a fork; mash it all up until there are no big chunks.
5. Then you can now use it right away, but for best flavor, I suggest you cover it with plastic wrap and refrigerate overnight.
6. This is when you heat the canola oil in a frying pan, and add the Fakin' Bacon.
7. After which you sauté until the pieces are brown and crispy.
8. Finally, you add the vegetables and stir-fry until they are tender.
9. After that, you add the tofu mixture and stir-fry until the tofu is heated through then you serves.

Nutritional value:
Amount per serving size: Each of 4 servings
Calories: 250
Carbohydrate: 9g
Dietary fiber: 4g
Protein: 24g

Tangy Grilled Salmon

Ingredients:
6 tablespoons of mustard
2 tablespoons of soy sauce
Sugar substitute to equal about 3 tablespoons of sugar
2 lb. salmon fillet
2 teaspoons of garlic powder
2 teaspoons of raw ginger root (grated)

Directions:
1. First, you mix the entire ingredients except for salmon.
2. Make sure the quantity of sweetener you want will vary with your desired taste.
3. However, do recognize that the heat from the ginger and mustard will mellow with cooking, thereby making the sweetness more prominent.
4. After that, you coat the salmon with about a third of the glaze.
5. Then you coat the top and sides, if the skin is on.
6. On the other hand, if the skin is off, I suggest you coat the whole thing, but use about half the glaze instead of a third.
7. After which you heat and oil the grill.
8. Furthermore, you cook the salmon skin side down for approximately 3-4 minutes, until you can view opaqueness about a third of the way up the side.
9. At this point, you turn the salmon.
10. After which if you lose the skin at this point, paint glaze on that side (or rather you can remove the skin easily with tongs if you do not want it).
11. Keep on cooking until salmon flakes, but is still darker inside than out this will take another 2-4 minutes.
12. Finally, you put the rest of the glaze on the salmon, before you serve.

Nutritional value:
Amount per serving size: Each serving
Calories: 238
Carbohydrate: 1g
Protein: 32g

Cranberry Walnut Cookies

Tips:
1. In this recipe, a mixture of whey protein powder and almond meal can be used in place of flour.
2. You will probably want to cut down the amount of sweetener in this recipe, that is If you are using the flavored protein powder (I recommend you use Designer brand Vanilla Praline or any liquid sweetener of your choice)
3. Preheat oven to a temperature of 375 F.

Note:
These drop cookies make a great healthy and nice Christmas cookie.

Ingredients:
2 cups of whey protein powder
8 oz. cream cheese (preferably low fat)
Sugar substitute equal to 3 cups sugar
2 teaspoons of baking soda
1 ¼ cups of chopped walnuts
3 cups of almond meal
1-cup (a stick) of butter
4 eggs
2 teaspoons of cinnamon
2 teaspoons of salt
2 cups of whole cranberries (fresh or frozen with no sugar added)

Directions:
1. First, you cream butter and cream cheese together until fluffy.
2. After which you add sweetener, cinnamon, and salt, and beat again.
3. After that, you add eggs, and beat until combined.
4. Then you add almond meal, protein powder, and baking soda and combine well.
5. At this point, you mix in cranberries and walnuts.
6. Finally, you drop by rounded spoonfuls onto an ungreased cookie sheet, or one covered with a silicone mat (Note: feel free to use any size, but avoid very large cookies).
7. Bake for about 7 to 9 minutes, until top is browning.
8. Make sure you cool before eating or store in a sealed container.

Nutritional value:
Amount per serving size: Each of 32 cookies

THE ATKINS DIET

Calories: 94
Fat: 5g
Carbohydrate: 1g
Dietary fiber: 1g
Protein: 4g

Dried Cranberries

Tips:
1. Do not be afraid to squish them down in the first phase (if not they will not dry the soluble fiber in them "gels" and retains water unless exposed to the air).
2. Preheat oven to a temperature of 200 F.

Ingredients:
2 Cups of sugar substitute of your choice (to taste)
2 bags of (24 oz.) fresh whole cranberries
1 Cup of water

Directions:
1. First, you put the cranberries in a large skillet.
2. After which you pick through to remove soft or brown ones.
3. If the sweetener is powdered, I suggest you dissolve in water.
4. After that, you pour over cranberries and stir.
5. At this point, you heat for approximately 4-5 minutes on medium high until cranberries pops.
6. Make sure you stir every minute or two.
7. When all seem popped, I suggest you turn off the burner and let them cool for 10 minutes.
8. Then you squish them down, using the back of a large spoon.

Note: do not be disturbed if it seems they are melding together.
9. Allow to cool for another 5 minutes or so.
10. Furthermore, you cover baking sheet with three layers of paper towels and a piece of parchment paper.
11. At this moment, you spread cranberries on the parchment. (Note: have faith they will mostly "individuate" again as they dry).
12. If there remain unpopped ones, I suggest you squish them down now.
13. Finally, you put in oven and turn heat down to 150 F.
14. After which in 2 to 4 hours, replace parchment and flip paper towels over. (It speeds up the process.)
15. Then you start checking it after 6 hours. (Note: The total time depends upon humidity and other factors).
16. You then separate, and store covered (I recommend a zip-type bags).

Nutritional value:
Amount per serving size: whole recipe
Carbohydrate: 25g

Garlic Parmesan Flax Seed Crackers

Tips:
1. This recipe is good with dips, spreads, or plain.

2. Heat the oven to a temperature of 400F.

Ingredients:
2 cups of flax seed meal
2/3 cup of Parmesan cheese (grated)
3 teaspoons of garlic powder
1 teaspoon of salt
1 cup of water

Directions:
1. First, you mix the entire ingredients together.
2. After which you spoon onto sheet pan covered with a silicone mat or greased parchment paper.
3. After that, you cover the mixture with a piece of parchment or waxed paper.
4. At this point, you even out the mixture to about 1/8 inches (I suggest you use a ruler, rolling pin or wine bottle).
Note: do not let it to be too thin around the edges or that part will overcook before the center firms up.
5. After you might have spread it out, then you remove the paper and go around the edges with your finger.
6. Push the thin part inwards to even it up.
7. Bake for approximately 15-18 minutes until the center is no longer soft.
8. If it starts to get more than a little brown around the edges, I suggest you remove from oven.
9. Allow it to cool completely (Note: it will continue to crisp up).
10. Then you can now break it into pieces.

Nutritional value:
Amount per serving size: whole recipe
Carbohydrate: 6g
Dietary fiber: 35g

Chopped Salad

Tips:
What I cherish the most in this recipe is the little bits of apple that give it a little sweet, crisp contrast to the salty bacon and creamy avocado.

Ingredients:
8 cups of romaine lettuce (chopped)
½ cup of green pepper (chopped)
½ cup of crumbled blue cheese
4 slices of cooked bacon (cut up into small bits)
1 cup of cooked chicken (chopped)
2 medium plum tomatoes (chopped)
½ cup of apple (chopped)
1 avocado (chopped)

Directions:
1. First, you toss ingredients together with an Italian or vinaigrette dressing (Makes one large meal-sized serving).

2. If you would like something less filling, I suggest you divide it or use fewer avocados.

Nutritional value:
Amount per serving size: Each serving (not counting dressing)
Calories: 484
Carbohydrate: 10g
Dietary fiber: 10g
Protein: 40g

Almond Pie Crust

TIPS:
It looks amazing with my No-Bake Cheesecake or Fresh Berry Pie.
Note: it works best for a 9" pie pan but if you have an 8" one, the crust will be a bit thicker, so you have to cut back on the ingredients.

Ingredients:
6 tablespoons of melted butter
3 cups of almond meal (or almond flour)
Artificial sweetener (equal to 6 tablespoons of sugar)

Directions:
1. First, you heat the oven to a temperature of 350 F.
2. After which you melt the butter (Note: you are to melt the butter in the microwave only if the pan is microwave safe).
3. After that, you mix the ingredients up in the pan and then use your fingertips to pat it into place.
4. At this point, you bake for approximately 10 minutes until the crust starts to brown.
5. Always check at every minute or so after 8 minute of baking, because once it begins to brown it goes quickly.

Nutritional value:
Amount per serving size: whole pie shell
Carbohydrate: 11g
Dietary fiber: 17g
Protein: 30g

Cherry Nut Cake

Ingredients:
2 cups of white sugar
2 teaspoons of baking soda
4 eggs
1 cup of chopped walnuts
4 cups of all-purpose flour
2 teaspoons of salt
1 ¼ cup of vegetable oil
Two (21-ounce) cans of cherry pie filling

Directions:
1. First, you place flour, sugar, salt, baking soda, oil, cherry pie filling, eggs, and chopped nuts in a 9x13 inch pan and mix thoroughly with a fork.
2. After which you bake in a preheated 350 degrees F (or 175 degrees C) oven for about 45 minutes.
3. Then you serve with whipped topping.

Nutritional value:
Amount per serving size: Each serving
Calories: 74
Fat: 5g
Carbohydrate: 6.8g
Dietary fiber: 4.6g
Protein: 1.8g

Conclusion

To lose weight is very easy if you know the process and how to go about it. That is the reason for this Book, to help you achieve your weight loss goal in No time. Get in shape while eating the foods you love. Take advantage of this healthy and delicious recipes provided for you in this book.
Remember, the only bad action you can take is no action at all.

THANK YOU

If you enjoyed this Book, please do not hesitate to Drop me a Review, it would be very Much Appreciated. Thanks!

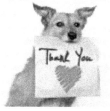

CPSIA information can be obtained
at www.ICGtesting.com
Printed in the USA
LVHW021108271220
675120LV00011B/450